CORE 4 OF WELLNESS

CORE 4 of Wellness

Nutrition | Physical Exercise | Stress Management | Spiritual Wellness

Kaushal B. Nanavati, MD

First Edition: April 2016
Library of Congress Control Number: 2016903598
CreateSpace Independent Publishing Platform
North Charleston, South Carolina
ISBN-13: 9781530256723
ISBN-10: 1530256720

1) Self-Help 2) Personal Growth 3) Happiness 4) Health, Mind, and Body 5) Body, Mind, and Spirit 6) Wellness 7) Stress Management 8) Spiritual Wellness 9) Motivational and Inspirational

Author speaking engagements may be addressed to core4ofwellness@gmail.com.

eBooks available from Internet retailers.

Cover Design: ebooklaunch.com

Cover Image: Deanna Benson and Divija Nanavati

Printed in the United States of America.

ACKNOWLEDGMENTS

Many thanks to the universe for inspiration, insight, and enlightenment! I would like to thank my parents and family for my early and foundational education and for teaching me the values of hard work and sacrifice. Through them I learned that when we give up what we think we *want*, we seem to get something even better—that which we actually *need*! I am thankful to my teachers and friends in school and in life who have taught me that my potential is limitless and that my duty is to give, not only to others but also to myself. All of these people helped me to understand myself well enough and honestly enough to recognize her when I met her as my partner in this life—my wife, who taught me to appreciate what we have and the true meaning of satisfaction and contentment. Together we are blessed with a son, who has reminded us of the joys of creation, growth, and the dynamic nature of life. My patients have been my extended family and these teachers of mine continue to inspire me to be the best version of myself as I guide them to do the same. Lastly, and just as importantly, I am thankful to you, the reader, for welcoming me into your life through the words on these pages in your search for contentment, peace, love, and wellness.

DISCLAIMER

This book provides an approach to wellness focusing on nutrition, physical exercise, stress management, and spiritual wellness. *CORE 4 of Wellness* is a guide for people interested in learning to manage their stress better and those seeking to have more balance and peace within their lives.

The methods described within this book are the author's personal thoughts. They are not intended to be a definitive set of instructions. You may discover there are other methods and materials to accomplish the same end result.

The discussion and guidance in this book do not replace sound medical advice from your physician or health care provider and do not substitute for medical therapeutic advice. The reader should regularly consult a physician or health care provider in matters relating to his or her health and particularly with respect to any symptoms that may require diagnosis or medical attention. It is recommended that you see your physician or health care provider before making any changes to your nutrition and physical exercise and activity regimen and for specific recommendations for you and your health and wellness.

Some names and identifying details have been changed to protect the privacy of individuals.

Although the author and publisher have made every effort to ensure that the information in this book was correct at press time, the author and publisher do not assume and hereby disclaim any liability to any party for any loss, damage, or disruption caused by errors or omissions, whether such errors or omissions result from negligence, accident, or any other cause.

The author and publisher advise readers to take full responsibility for their safety and know their limits. The information contained within this book is strictly for educational purposes. If you wish to apply ideas contained in this book, you are taking full responsibility for your actions.

Cover Image Description

In writing *CORE 4 of Wellness*, I wanted the cover image to capture the holistic approach of the book. The fork and spoon represent nutrition. The footprints represent physical exercise and the journey of life. The lit candle represents self-awareness, and the glow signifies the creation of an enlightened presence, addressing stress management and spiritual wellness. The union of the four cores of wellness in this image completes the circle of life.

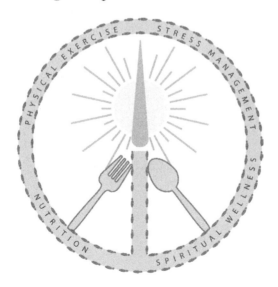

INTRODUCTION

If you think of health care as a tree, think of the trunk as disease prevention, the branches as disease management, and the leaves as innovations, some of which become new branches and others of which fall by the wayside. The roots of the tree are wellness promotion. My goal is to help people strengthen their roots of health and wellness. *CORE 4 of Wellness* provides a holistic approach to wellness of the mind, body, and spirit in simple, understandable language. The book provides an approach to wellness focusing on nutrition, physical exercise, stress management, and spiritual wellness. Included in this book are stress management exercises to help the readers define and refine their approaches to handling stress. Also presented are simple examples to help affect positive changes in nutrition and physical exercise routines. The chapters are short and focused, addressing each core with simple examples and points to ponder.

The purpose of this book is to allow the reader an opportunity to reflect on his or her own values, goals, and vision of a peaceful life. Ask yourself a simple question: "Am I con*tent* with my *con*tent?" If your answer is a resounding yes, try to understand why so that you can always hold onto it. If your answer is no, then let's explore some of the possibilities of why your answer is no and how it can become yes. Are you not satisfied because of your job or not having a job? Is it your boss, spouse, finances, or maybe some other reason? If you're not sure *and* you want to feel different, then it's worth taking some time to figure it out. How are you going to solve a problem if you don't know what it is? How are you going to get somewhere if you don't know where you're going? After all, it is *your* life!

My intention with this book is not to say, "This is the only way." I am simply suggesting that the pearls in this book can guide you to achieve peace for yourself, based on *your* philosophy and *your* goals. People should feel inspired to live healthier lives with greater peace and acceptance.

As a family and integrative physician, I work with people of all ages and backgrounds. Along the way, I have come upon some core themes about finding peace in life. This book is a culmination of insights based on these pearls gathered from my own life experiences.

We may not always be happy, but we can learn to be at peace with any given situation.

Think about it! I will use this "think about it" phrase throughout this book. This phrase has great value in guiding one to a more peaceful life.

Think about it! It makes so much sense. Most of us know right from wrong. We know what we need and what we want, and when we are struggling to make a decision, all we have to do is make the choice that brings peace. Think about the consequences of your actions, and if they are also grounded in your peace, then you are on the right path!

Think about it! Throughout this book I have used this phrase to bring forth a pause. This was intentional and meant to be a time to reflect about and inspect your values and your goals.

TABLE OF CONTENTS

Strengthen Your Fort

Our health behaviors can be interesting. So many times we hear people say, "If it ain't broke, don't fix it" or "Why get a regular checkup when I'm feeling fine?"

I have heard these statements over the years, but I have an approach to understanding health, and the idea is simple:

Strengthen your fort!
If your fort is strong enough, you have to worry less about
the invaders coming in!

In many cases, by the time we are able to detect disease, the disease has already progressed. While diagnostic technology and screening tests are getting better at detecting disease and even disease potential (through genetic testing), we know that an ounce of prevention really is worth a pound of cure. The best way to avoid disease is to strengthen the body, mind, and spirit.

A *strong body* allows us to physically function with greater ease and less *disease*.

A *strong mind* helps to reduce detracting thoughts such as doubt, fear, and greed while promoting an attitude of gratitude, the ability to focus, and an understanding of needs versus wants and providing the determination to overcome obstacles.

A strong spirit allows one to understand concepts such as satisfaction, contentment, peace, and love of self and others providing the courage and calm to see life as a beautiful journey with each experience a destination unto itself.

"The joy is in the journey" can mean that every moment of your journey is an end to itself as well as a starting point to moving forward all at the same time. Every ending is a new beginning!

Strengthening and balancing the body, mind, and spirit allows us to strengthen our fort, to build lives grounded in contentment and peace. These feelings are not as remote as one might think. Our ultimate goal, whether to climb the corporate ladder, become a billionaire, invent something, or whatever, is to experience contentment and peace.

If we wait to experience satisfaction, joy, contentment, and peace only when we achieve goals we have set, then these feelings seem to be like the dangling fruit of a tree that can only be tasted by those who can reach them. Some people are able to maintain these feelings and use them as guiding principles while setting and achieving new goals. Others seem to never be able to hold onto these feelings. There was even a study published in 2012 that showed that people who are more "self-centered," meaning those who "try to maximize pleasures and to avoid displeasures," had more fluctuating happiness.[1] If they had pleasure, they were happy, and if they didn't, then they weren't happy. People who were more "selfless," those who had the ability to "deal with whatever comes [their] way in life," had more durable happiness. These people seemed to have the inner resources to deal with success and failure, and their sense of worth and value wasn't tied to individual situations as much as it was to their sense of self-worth. Rather

---

1 M. Dambrun et al., "Measuring Happiness: From Fluctuating Happiness to Authentic Durable Happiness," *Front Psychol* 3 no. 16 (2012).

than saying things like, "I didn't get this, so..." "I'm no good," or "I feel horrible," these "selfless" people may think, "I didn't get this, but I'm still good; it just didn't work out this time. I'm good with who I am."

Self-centered people tend to attach their happiness to things, people, and situations outside of themselves. If they get the goal, they are happy, and if they don't, then they are not. So happiness fluctuates for them like a yo-yo, coming and going, sometimes in their grasp and sometimes spiraling away. They give control of their happiness to things outside of themselves, and so they never have control over their happiness. Their happiness is dependent on the things in their lives, their wants, and whether they can get these things or not.

Selfless people are different. These people are satisfied with themselves and are well rooted in their sense of self-worth. Their fort is strong, and so they do not let the external things and wants take away their sense of happiness, even when they may not have been able to get those things. Satisfaction, contentment, and peace are the fertile soil in which they are rooted—their fortress—and these are the ingredients that help them to sustain their happiness. Love of self is their nourishment that they imbibe, with which they water their "plants"—their souls, their bodies, and their minds.

So how can a person maintain peace and contentment and still strive to be his or her best each day? In order to achieve this, I believe we each need a strong foundation of wellness. I have termed this foundation the *CORE 4 of Wellness.* The idea is that wellness of body, mind, and spirit can be grounded in the four cores of nutrition, physical exercise, stress management, and spiritual wellness.

Own what's yours, and let go of the rest! Why wait for someone else or something else to change before you can feel happy?

Either change something about what's stressing you, or change how you're looking at it.

When you go to bed at night, your body will be able to relax into sleep if you can allow your mind to relax first. Look back at your day with gratitude for all that went well and even for that which did not go well, knowing that the lessons of today will help to strengthen your fort tomorrow!

Happiness truly is an inside job!

PART 1

THE FIRST CORE OF WELLNESS:

NUTRITION

HOW TO FORM HEALTHY HABITS

Before we talk about nutrition, we need to talk about how to form healthy habits. We may know what is healthy or good for us, but we may not know how to implement the healthy behavior in our daily lives or are just not able to motivate ourselves to make the change.

Why do we struggle with adopting and maintaining healthy habits? Some people just never learned any better due to the patterns they have seen in their own lives among parents, siblings, or friends.

While medical science continues to advance in the detection and prevention of disease, we make less time for self-care, whether it be taking time to prepare healthy food, physical exercise and activity, or destressing. People are stressed about finances and jobs, and all of this impacts the choices we make.

The idea behind establishing any habit is repetition. Whether the habit is good or bad, the more you repeat a pattern of behavior, the more engrained it gets, and over time this habit becomes a more natural instinct. While the old habit may not completely go away, the newer habit becomes the go-to more readily.

Most of us change our behavior for two main reasons:

1) The reward for change is greater than the current behavior.
2) The risk of not changing the behavior is thought to be too great!

Otherwise, we don't change.

Think about it! Forming a habit takes an average of sixty-six days, according to research published by Phillippa Lally and colleagues.[2] They note that in order to successfully create a new habit, repetition of the habit within the same environment on a consistent basis is important. In other words, the more regularly you do something, the more likely it is to become automatic. The sixty-six days is an average, and obviously this time frame varies for people depending on their commitment to the new habit, how strongly they feel about the old habit they are trying to change, how regularly they practice the new habit, and so on.

For example, people who smoke cigarettes with their morning coffee, during work breaks, or after meals are used to this pattern. In order to break from the old pattern and establish a new pattern, smokers are going to have to actively change their behavior. So let's look at the steps needed to change behavior.

1) First, you have to have the interest and commitment to change. No matter how much friends, family, or the health care provider want you to change, if you are not committed and the need for change doesn't come from within, you are not likely to successfully form the new habit.

2) Next, you have to set the stage. Be specific about the change or new habit you wish to form, and define the setting. If you are going to eat oatmeal and fruit in the morning instead of drinking coffee and having a cigarette, then be specific with that plan, and stick to it daily until it becomes automatic. The old habit doesn't just go, but the new one will become stronger.

---

2 P. Lally, C. H. M. van Jaarsveld, H. H. W. Potts, and J. Wardle, "How Are Habits Formed: Modelling Habit Formation in the Real World," *European Journal of Social Psychology* 40 (2010): 998–1009.

3) Actively support yourself by telling yourself, "I am making a positive change for myself and am making a healthier choice." You can reinforce your behavior by feeling good about it. Understand that the healthier choice is the real treat for your body, mind, and spirit. I am amused when I think that we (including myself, for some of these) have considered ice cream, cake, soda, cigarettes, alcohol, screen time, and late-night clubbing as rewards for "good" behavior or as rites of passage! In reality, vegetables, fruits, nuts, healthy foods, adequate sleep, maintaining lower stress, and regular physical exercise are the *real* treats for the body, mind, and spirit. Not many people think of broccoli or asparagus as a treat, and yet these can take care of the body much better than processed packaged foods! *If you want others to be kind to you, then start by being kind to yourself!* Eat healthy foods that nourish your body rather than fatty, greasy, fried, processed foods that are harmful to the body and can cause inflammation.

4) The last part is creating the habit. Once you've committed to the positive change, form the habit. Change one thing at a time, if it is easier for you, and stick with it! You are resetting a foundation that is grounded in healthier habits, and as you do this, you create a healthier future for yourself. When parents do this, they give the priceless gifts of good health and good habits to their children. In fact, with children, when we want them to eat healthier foods, if we just take away everything that they like and replace it with food that we want them to eat, food that they may not like or have tasted before, they are more likely to reject it or rebel. However, if we simply add a little amount of the food we want them to have with the food they like to have, then

over time, they will accept the little bit we give and will associate the tastes together as the new item slowly blends in. Over time, we can increase the portion of the "good" food we want them to have and reduce the portion of the "not so good" food we want them to reduce. Since they have started to associate the tastes, it becomes much more manageable.

Remember to consult your physician or health care provider before making changes that may affect or interfere with your health conditions or health care.

Start with yourself, and be selfish with self-care, self-love, and self-respect! Create an environment of healthier habits for your body, mind, and spirit using *CORE 4 of Wellness*, and enjoy every day of your life! Be thankful and be at peace!

After all, at any given moment in life, you have two choices. You can choose to be at peace, or you can make the other choice, but the choice is always yours. Don't point the finger elsewhere!

Patience and persistence lead to healthier habits!

HEALTHY EATING RECOMMENDATIONS

One of the most common questions I am asked is, "What should I be eating?" My feeling is that food should be flavorful and fun while also being healthy. After all, this is the fuel we provide our bodies. Food is used for celebrations, gatherings, and ceremonies, and many of us plan our vacations around food!

Below is a general summary of healthy eating recommendations. Remember to consult your physician or health care provider before making changes, as the recommendations may vary depending on your health condition(s), allergies, or current therapies.

Try to spread your food over four to six meals per day. The meals can be any combination of breakfast, midmorning snack, lunch, midafternoon snack, dinner, and an evening snack (though try not to eat within a couple of hours of bedtime).

1) Vegetables: have seven to nine servings of vegetables daily. Eat a variety, or rainbow, of vegetables.

    One serving of vegetables equals one measuring cup of raw vegetables/salad greens or half a measuring cup of cooked vegetables.

    This sounds like a daunting task, but if you have a decent-sized salad (two to three measuring cups) for lunch and for dinner, you've already consumed five to six servings. Then if you snack on some carrot sticks, broccoli, cucumbers, or the like, then you can easily get to seven or more servings. Avoid creamy salad dressings. Instead, try using lemon or lime along with a dash of black pepper and a dash of salt or salt substitute. This tastes really good with steamed broccoli or chopped carrots and cucumbers or corn.

2) Fruits: have one to two servings per day. Eat a variety, or rainbow, of fruits.

One serving of fruit equals a small fruit such as an apple, banana, or orange; one cup of berries; or two tablespoons dried fruit.

For diabetics I would recommend one serving earlier in the day or split into a half serving twice per day.

3) Protein: enjoy protein with each meal.

One serving of protein equals one-third measuring cup cooked lentils, beans, or peas; three ounces of fish; or a palm-sized serving of lean meat.

The recommendation is to get at least 0.36 grams of protein per pound. So for a 150-pound person, the amount of protein needed is at least 54 grams per day—split over four to six meals. Protein can be obtained from multiple sources.

a. Beans, legumes, and lentils should be the primary source of protein unless you have certain health conditions that impact the absorption or digestion of these.

b. If you're going to eat meat, then eat fish, turkey, or chicken in that order of preference. I'm not talking about fried fish or chicken! (I know that some of your mouths are watering right now thinking about fried fish and fried chicken, but *no fried food!*) Try to get organic, grass-fed meat whenever possible.

   c. Avoid processed meats. They can be high in salt and have pro-inflammatory potential in the body.

   d. When meat is well done or cooked at high temperatures, chemicals known as heterocyclic amines (HCA) and polycyclic aromatic hydrocarbons are formed that can be associated with the development of certain cancers. More information can be obtained on this at the following website:

      http://www.cancer.gov/about-cancer/causes-prevention/risk/diet/cooked-meats-fact-sheet

4) Grains: whole grains are better (oats, barley, quinoa, etc.).

    Some people have sensitivity or intolerance to certain grains, so please eat the healthy foods that your body can handle!

5) Nuts: walnuts and almonds are better for cholesterol than peanuts and cashews. Eat the healthier nuts more regularly and the other nuts, which are still a decent source of protein, less often. Pistachios, pecans, and brazil nuts are also healthy. In fact, two brazil nuts per day may give you all the chromium and selenium you need for an entire day! Remember to eat nuts in moderation.

6) Dairy: primarily enjoy plain yogurt or yogurt smoothies.

    You can add fruit, vegetables, or honey to plain yogurt to make a delicious smoothie. Greek yogurt has more protein per serving compared to regular yogurt.

7) Drink: have water as your primary drink.

    Limit juice. (It's better to eat the fruit than to just have juice, as eating the fruit gives you soluble and insoluble fiber that, among other health benefits, can help with bow-el movement regularity—keeping your intestines clean!)

Vegetarian eating has tremendous health benefits, but if you're going to eat meat, then the meat should be added *after* you've placed the vegetables, beans, grains, and fruit on your plate and placed the water and yogurt on the side.

Try not to eat bread, rice, potato, pasta, and cheese after lunch. Carbohydrates are a great source of fuel, and you can have these earlier in your day when you have a greater chance of using them as energy. You should avoid loading up on carbohydrates at night when you will be less active and store them as starch. The example I like to give is that we fuel up our car before we go on a long jour-ney and not when it's parked in the garage. The same goes for the body.

The above is a broad summary of a healthy eating pattern. Everyone's caloric needs are different, and you should create your meal plan in conjunction with your health care provider based on your health conditions, allergies, and other needs. For more information, you can refer to Harvard University's evi-dence-based "Healthy Eating Plate" (web link: http://www.hsph. harvard.edu/nutritionsource/) or to the US government's "My Plate" (web link: http://www.choosemyplate.gov/). They have sev-eral resources and tools to help guide you to healthier eating and healthier living!

Simple ways to get creative with your food and remain healthy include the following:

a) Steam broccoli. Then add a pinch of salt or salt substitute and black pepper with fresh lime squeezed on top.

b) Chop some carrots and cucumbers and add a pinch of salt or salt substitute and black pepper with fresh lime squeezed on top.

c) Roast corn. Then put a little salt or salt substitute and black pepper in a bowl and dip a lime in the mix and rub on the corn. *Delicious…and no butter required!*

Bon appétit!

HALF THE SIZE TO HALF YOUR SIZE

The title of this chapter should be shouted from the mountaintops and placed on every billboard. Obesity is becoming a major epidemic in many parts of the world. The amount of calories we consume has gone up steadily over the past few decades while the level of activity has declined. Food portions in restaurants are bigger, especially in the United States. Buffets test the resolve in even the best of us because we feel bad if we don't go for seconds. For crying out loud, it's a buffet—of course I have to get my money's worth! One plate only? Pshh! You're not eating your money's worth! I know many of you reading this have thought it just as much as I can admit I have in the past.

So the new motto, a mantra to be repeated many times before entering a restaurant or sitting down for a meal is, "Half the size to half *your* size." Ask for *half a portion* at a restaurant, order a small plate, or order one item and split it with another person. "What?" you say. "Why would I do that?" Well, the fact is that some restaurants may discount your meal if you ask for a smaller portion, while others may not. At the end of the day, the reality is simple. By reducing your portion size, you will still get to eat the food that you like, but you won't overdo it. Your calories are better controlled, and realistically, the portion was too big anyway. Think about how we are brought up. We are told to finish the food on our plate from childhood. In fact, we are not just told—it is demanded in many cases. Statements such as, "There are people starving in the world, and you want to just waste your food?" are repeated over and over again. The reality is, the food that I don't finish is not directly going to feed someone starving ten thousand miles away, or even if they were in my back yard. More importantly, by my finishing and overeating, I am ultimately going to harm my own body. Instead, we should take smaller portions and teach children to do the same. It is more prudent to take some more later on than to overload your plate and then waste it. By doing this, we are less likely to overeat.

If you are trying to lose some weight and are nervous about an upcoming gathering, try this approach. I call it the *tablespoon rule*. You may like the entire menu and want to eat all the items, but make a deal with yourself. Allow yourself to have a tablespoon serving of each meal item that you want, and that is it! So you can still indulge in the foods of your choosing but in much smaller quantities, and by having the choice, you can feel in control and enjoy every bite. Try it out the next time you have a family gathering or picnic.

Think about how this principle can apply in other aspects of your life. For example, if you are someone who says yes to everything and everyone, you are likely to overload your plate and get overwhelmed. However, if you are disciplined and understand your limits, then you can still help others without creating greater stress in your own life.

Savor the moment and savor the morsel!

PART 2

THE SECOND CORE OF WELLNESS: PHYSICAL EXERCISE

EXERCISE: SCHEDULE IT

While I do encourage you to exercise and discuss ways to initiate this below, engaging in vigorous physical activity or exercise without proper preparation can lead to potential injury or health consequences. Please consult with a health care provider prior to engaging in strenuous or vigorous physical activity.

There is a difference between physical activity and physical exercise. Activity can refer to getting up from a chair, walking to the kitchen, opening up the cupboard, and grabbing some cookies. *That*, my friends, is not exercise!

The definition of exercise I am referring to is defined by the World Health Organization (WHO) as "a subcategory of physical activity that is planned, structured, repetitive, and purposeful in the sense that the improvement or maintenance of one or more components of physical fitness is the objective."[3]

For those who are inactive, the data from the WHO suggests, "Physical inactivity (lack of physical activity) has been identified as the fourth leading risk factor for global mortality (6% of deaths globally). Moreover, physical inactivity is estimated to be the main cause for approximately 21–25% of breast and colon cancers, 27% of diabetes and approximately 30% of ischemic heart disease

---

3 World Health Organization, Global Strategy on Diet, Physical Activity and Health (2016) http://www.who.int/dietphysicalactivity/pa/en/index.html

burden."[3] We also know that exercise can improve depression, relieve stress, and enhance an overall sense of well-being.

Most of us live on schedules. We get up with an alarm, eat breakfast (maybe), go to work, eat lunch around noon (although some people skip lunch), and then go back home when work is done. This is the routine.

Once home, most of us are too tired or too busy—tending to kids, working around the house, cooking, and so on—that exercise is the last thing on our minds. For many of us, if we don't put it on our schedules, it won't happen. This is why I want you to *make it a daily appointment.* In fact, according to the United States Office of Disease Prevention and Health Promotion (ODPHP), "It has been estimated that people who are physically active for approximately 7 hours a week have a 40 percent lower risk of dying early than those who are active for less than 30 minutes a week."[4] Think of it this way: one hour is roughly 4 percent of your day, and 30 minutes in a week is a little more than 4 minutes a day, not even 0.1%. In other words, bump up your investment from nearly nothing in a day to just over 4 percent a day, and you get a 40 percent gain! Are you with me so far? Who wouldn't want that kind of investment! *Think about it!*

Exercise is not a want—it is a need *for wellness!*

---

4 Physical Activity Guidelines, Chapter 2: Physical Activity Has Many Health Benefits (2016)
http://health.gov/paguidelines/guidelines/chapter2.aspx

Simple Recommendations for Exercise

The current recommendations say to get a total of two and a half hours of exercise per week. Many people undershoot the mark, but why not aim higher, strive to be better, take the time to improve your health, and reduce the risk of illness?

Here are some simple recommendations on exercise:

1. Aim for sixty minutes of moderate intensity exercise on most days, even if it's simply walking at a brisk pace. Moderate intensity means you're going hard enough where you can speak in small sentences but are not going so hard that you will pass out or so slow that you can have long-winded conversations.
2. Another approach is to get a pedometer and walk
    a. 10,000 steps per day to roughly maintain weight; or
    b. 12,000-14,000 steps per day to burn more calories.
3. If you're going to lift weights and do cardiovascular exercise as part of a workout, then after you have stretched and done your warm-up, do the weights first, and then do the cardio. Weight lifting can boost the rate at which you burn calories (your metabolic rate).
4. During the cardio portion of your workout, try to go for longer duration. You can also do an interval workout (as

opposed to a constant pace), as this will lead to greater calorie burning and a higher metabolism for a longer time after you have finished the exercise. An interval workout refers to alternating speeds between a fast pace for a brief period and then a moderate pace for a brief period. An example would be to go at a fast pace for one minute followed by going at a moderate pace for two minutes, and then repeat the pattern for the duration of your workout.

5. Be sure to stretch after the workout (as well as before), as this is important to prevent injury. Also, get at least ten to fifteen grams of protein (and not more than twenty to twenty-five grams) within thirty minutes of finishing the workout. This will help with muscle recovery afterward. People with kidney disease or diabetes should be careful not to overload on protein.

6. Be sure your exercise is something you enjoy and can do regularly.

7. Tai chi, yoga, and meditation are excellent forms of mind, body, and spirit strengthening and balancing exercises. Please choose what you enjoy!

If you want others to respect you, then start by respecting yourself! Treat your body with respect by building a strong foundation with regular physical exercise. Go for a walk. Go to the gym. Play a game. Do whatever you can to strengthen your heart, improve your stamina, and improve your flexibility.

Make exercise a daily appointment, and you will be on your path to a sound body and sound mind to accompany an invigorated spirit!

GOLDEN LIGHT MEDITATION

It is well known that deep, slow abdominal breathing can do everything from reducing anxiety, averting anxiety attacks, and reducing blood pressure to increasing focus and concentration. It can happen in as little as ten to twelve minutes per day of deep breathing. In fact, one deep breath can make a difference, and thus the saying "Take a deep breath!"

This simple breathing exercise that I call "golden light meditation" is a way to help bring the calm into your life so that you can heal and be content!

1. Get yourself in a comfortable and relaxed position whether you are sitting, standing, or lying down. Breathe in through the nose for a count of five to ten seconds, and then breathe out through the mouth for a count of five to ten seconds. Continue breathing and when you start out, you may not be able to take as deep a breath, so you can breathe in as long as is comfortable and breathe out as long as you can. Over time try to extend it out a bit longer. The five to ten second time frame is simply a guide.

2. Pay attention to your body. When you breathe in, your shoulders should not rise, but your abdomen should push

out. Think of your belly as a balloon. As you breathe in, let the balloon fill up.

3. As you breathe out through your mouth, the abdomen (balloon) empties.
4. Slowly continue breathing in and breathing out.
5. Close your eyes, and envision a golden light on the top of your head.
6. With each breath, feel your body slowly getting soaked by this golden light like a sponge. Every time you breathe in feel the light soaking the area of focus and when you breathe out bring the light further down. First let the light fill your head and slowly continue bringing it down into your neck, then to your shoulders and arms down to your fingers, chest, abdomen, pelvis, and legs down to your toes.
7. Then bring the golden light slowly back up in the reverse order soaking each of those areas as it reaches the top of your head.
8. While doing this, don't try to block thoughts out of your mind. Instead, allow them to come in a free-flowing manner. If a thought appears, let it! Wonder why it is there, and then as it goes, another thought will come. This is your mind's way of decluttering, and it's perfect! Every time your mind drifts, just bring it back to the golden light and visualize where the light is in your body and continue to take it further.
9. Make a commitment to yourself for sixty-six days. Let this meditation help you increase your physical, mental, and spiritual wellness.

Inhale peace, exhale stress!

PART 3

THE THIRD CORE OF WELLNESS: STRESS MANAGEMENT

A Five-Step Approach for Stress Management

What is stress? According to a definition in *Merriam-Webster's Dictionary*, stress is "a physical, chemical, or emotional factor that causes bodily or mental tension and may be a factor in disease causation."

Stress is a part of most of our lives. Oh, what am I saying? Stress is a part of all of our lives. From the instant we are conceived until our last breath, we experience stress in many different ways. There are positive stressors such as learning to ride a bicycle, the first kiss, getting a driver's license, and getting accepted into college. Then there are negative stressors such as falling off of that bicycle for the first time, breaking up from a relationship, suffering illness and disease, and so on.

There are stresses in life that we can do something about...
and then there are stresses that we cannot control.

Understanding this concept is crucial to understanding which stresses to take ownership of and which ones to let go.

Know what's really yours—own it, deal with it, and let
go of the rest!

Remember that there is only one person that can truly balance your life…and that, my friend, is *you*!

Following is a five-step approach to stress management that can help you sort out and prioritize your stressors.

1. Take a sheet of paper, and make a list of all the things that give you stress, tension, worry, anxiety, or concern, from the smallest, meaningless ones to the things that are always on your mind. Feel free to use more than one sheet if needed.

2. Then on a second sheet of paper, make two columns. Label the first column "Things I can do something about" and the second column "Things that I cannot control."

3. Now take the list that you first made, and sort out the list into the two columns on the second sheet. For example, I can control what I'm going to wear or eat or phone calls I'm going to make. I cannot control other people's actions or reactions to something I've done. Even if you have eight pages of stressors, when you sort the stressors into the two columns, you may find that only one page worth of stressors are things that you can do something about. The other seven pages of stressors, while they may be in your life, are not things that you may be the primary person to resolve.

4. The stresses you cannot control will remain on the list until someone else takes care of them, as you can do nothing about them. An example would be worrying about a test after you've taken it. Once you've taken the test, you have the stress of waiting for the results, but you have no control over it at that point. Sweat it before the test, and study to make yourself as well prepared as possible. But once you've taken the test, it is no longer in your hands, so move on! Look at this column of stressors you cannot control and say to

yourself, "Yep, these things are on my plate, but somebody or something else is going to get them off; I am not the one who can solve these."

5. The stresses you can do something about are truly yours to deal with! So take one item at a time, and make a written action plan to get it resolved and off your list. Then when it is done, cross it off your list. Literally take a permanent marker and cross it off, as this act of physically crossing it off will feel *really* good and give you a sense of control over your stressors, knowing that you are actively taking care of the things you can do something about. As each new issue comes up, just ask yourself if that issue is something you can do anything about or if it goes in the other column. This exercise will allow you to understand stress and deal with the things you can do something about instead of worrying about things that are out of your control.

There may also be some stresses for which you can take care of part of the problem, and the rest really belongs to someone else. That's OK! Just handle your part because that's the only part you can control.

This approach will work in your personal and professional life and will help you better prioritize your responsibilities and classic to-do lists.

> *When you stress about a stressor, you have two problems.*
> *When you take care of the stress, you have no problems!*

Think about those two previous statements. You can use the same energy to worry about something or to take care of it. It is the same energy, and it is simply a matter of how you use that energy.

One plus one is two, while one minus one is zero. They are the same numbers, but when added, they grow, and when subtracted, they are no more. The same goes for stress. The same energy, when added to your stress in the form of worry, only increases your stress. Yet when that energy is used to take away your stress, your stress is resolved!

In the next few chapters, I will share further thoughts on dealing with stress and how to create better balance and buffers in different areas of your life.

Don't be distressed, become destressed!

CREATING YOUR BALANCE IN LIFE

Do you feel that your life is balanced? I want to discuss the concept of balance as it applies in our daily lives. If you want to live a balanced life, who is going to do it for you? *No one else can balance your life for you; you have to do it for yourself!* You have to look to the person in the mirror (yourself) to achieve balance in your life, whether it is emotional, financial, spiritual, or otherwise.

Feeling unsettled, restless, bored, confused, or overwhelmed means that you are not feeling balanced—like you can't handle what's on your plate. Oftentimes this happens when we feel stressed. Stress in its various forms is a natural part of life, and when we understand how to deal with it, we are able to navigate a path through it that allows us to maintain our balance.

Feeling stressed is an emotional response that is not a comfortable feeling, nor is it necessary to hold onto. This emotional response can lead to mental and physical harm if not dealt with properly. We can use the five-step approach to stress management to address aspects of stress and balance related to our finances, emotions, relationships, health, and work.

A perfect example is that of a surfer who is balancing his or her body on a surfboard that also needs to be balanced on the ever-changing waves of the ocean. This dynamic process defines the journey of life so vividly! In the ocean of life, you have to continually adjust and optimize your relationship with these waves so that there is harmony and rebalancing as needed.

Emotional Balance

You have to feel the feelings you feel! There's no way around that. If you're angry or sad, mad or glad, or even at peace, you have feelings. There's nothing wrong with feelings. Accept them, acknowledge them, and work with them, but don't let negative feelings and emotions dictate your actions.

There is a common thread among all world philosophies and religions. Negative emotions such as anger, frustration, greed, lust, and fear are grounded in ignorance and attachment. "Ignorance" simply means a lack of knowledge or awareness. "Attachment" refers to our connection with things and people in our lives but also to an expectation we have of them based on what *we* want or need—not necessarily based on what *they* want or need. When things don't go according to what we were expecting, then we feel those negative feelings. Many of us are then disappointed, and, when we really think about it, sometimes we are disappointed in ourselves for having high hopes or expectations.

One day when I was feeling some resentment and a sense of hopelessness, I had a thought that was simply enlightening and helped me to find a new sense of emotional balance. Expect the most out of yourself, and expect very little from others. In this way, you are less likely to be disappointed. After all, the only person you can have any potential to control is yourself, and even that is not so easy. In expecting the most out of yourself, expect yourself to be more kind, to be more warm, to be more giving and forgiving, and to be more accepting of others and of yourself. This requires discipline, focus, planning, and creating healthy patterns of be-havior. As we slowly do this, we start to feel greater contentment, self-worth, satisfaction, and a sense of peace. If others in our life behave in the same manner, then soon there is peace within our relationships.

Perfection Is a Well-Balanced State

Let me first define what I mean by "perfection." This refers to peace in life. A healthy mind without a healthy body or spirit doesn't lead to peace. So if perfection is defined as peace, then peace is attained when you are in a well-balanced state. A well-balanced state refers to balance of mind, body, and spirit – find-ing *your* balance in relationships, finances, emotions, health, school or work performance, fun and joy in life, and peace and contentment!

Think about it! People sometimes put all of their energy into one thing—let's say work, for example. Then their home life suffers. I've known people who felt that "achieving something" referred only to getting recognition from the outside world. They forget that creating a happy home is one of the greatest achievements one can have. Figuring out how to do both is an art of give and take. When your peace becomes the deciding factor on what you give and what you take then you start to build a life that seems more balanced.

Others might spend all of their time in recreation and not pay attention to their work, so their work suffers. A boy who comes home from school and plays all evening, not getting his home-work done, would enjoy the perfect playtime but not have a per-fect school record. Think about a seesaw. It can only be perfectly balanced when there is enough weight or value on both sides.

Otherwise it tips to one side or the other. Common language and phrases that have been used to express this wisdom include "Get your ducks in a row" or "Put a nickel in every basket."

Acceptance and forgiveness lead to contentment and peace!

EVERY RELATIONSHIP HAS AN OPTIMAL DISTANCE

Once a friend of mine said something so deep and so profound that it has stayed with me and guided my relationships to this day. He said, "Every relationship has an optimal distance."

Think about it! Every relationship has an optimal distance. Remember that one person who kept annoying you, and it just seemed like he or she was invading your space? This is an example of the adage "too close for comfort."

On the other hand, think of those times when you felt an instant connection with someone and the friendship or relationship just seemed right.

Examine your own life, and think about this notion of optimal distance. Think about the people whom you are in relationship with. Do all of these relationships seem in balance? On some days, do you feel a disconnect, or conversely, do you feel flustered and constricted, as if they are invading your space? Do you feel like they have too much control or are too controlling or that you don't have enough say in things? If so, you are experiencing a sense of imbalance. There is no sense of harmony. Over time relationships settle into what one may think of as a natural balance based on each side's strengths and weaknesses, hopes and wishes, dreams, goals, and expectations. You develop a natural balance, and on some days you feel like you can talk about anything. On others, it seems as if you—or they—need space. The concept of optimal distance is illustrated in this diagram:

Too Far (you don't quite connect)

<----------------------   ----------------------->

Too Close (you can feel friction or constricted)

>>>==<<<

Just Right (it works)

☺----------------------☺

Every one of your relationships has that right distance or comfort zone. If you venture out of that comfort zone, things can get uncomfortable or awkward, and the relationship just doesn't quite seem to work. When we reach the right balance in a relationship, it seems easy. How often do we hear the phrase, "We're struggling to find the right balance," "I just don't get him (or her)," or "I wish she'd tell me what she wants!"

The relationship between a boss and an employee has a different balance than the relationship between a husband and wife or a parent and child.

So with each of your relationships, think about what the *optimal distance* is, and try to see if you can achieve it. Not everyone in your life needs to be your best friend, and that is OK. With some people, maintaining a cordial distance is a good thing—for you and for them. With others, it's OK to let your guard down, as this may actually help the relationship blossom and grow.

In nature, the planets and the sun have found an optimal distance, and the planets maintain their orbit. If they were to get out of that "comfort zone" in the relationship, the planet would spin out of orbit or be drawn in too close and be consumed by the more dominant celestial body. In nature, electrons and protons find their optimal distance for balance and coexistence. This is true in our relationships as well.

You may also find that even with the same person on different days, the optimal distance is different, either closer or farther. We can't usually adjust the other person's position, but we can adjust our own. If you're feeling some sort of disconnect with the other person, *think about it!* Are you too close or not quite connecting? Then adjust your position to create that optimal distance, and both of you will feel more comfortable.

Once we understand optimal distance, we are able to journey with a greater sense of peace and contentment.

Find your optimal distance and you will find peace!

The Joy Is in the Journey

As we journey through life, we share our paths with various individuals along the way. What we realize is that we share part of the journey with some people, and then their path may take them in a different direction while ours may go in another. We can think of this in two ways.

One approach is to regret that we are no longer together with those individuals. The other approach is to value the shared journey for what it was and for the impact it had on our lives. If it was a positive experience, then relish it, and if it was a negative experience, then take solace in the fact that you are now journeying in a different direction.

One way to understand relationships is to use the analogy of a ladder. The two posts of a ladder are separate pieces in and of themselves. Yet they are connected and remain joined by the rungs of the ladder. Without the rungs, the two posts would fall apart. In other words, the two posts need the rungs to keep them together. In a relationship between two individuals, these rungs represent commitment, compromise, honesty, forgiveness, communication, acceptance, love, caring, availability, shared goals, mutual respect, and trust.

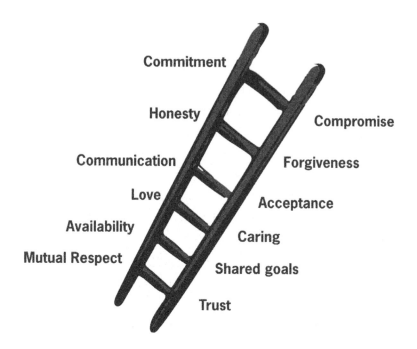

Relationships are like a ladder

These rungs allow for a stronger relationship and help to strengthen the bond between the two individuals. Yet there are times in our lives when these may be in place, and still we journey in different directions; for instance, when you moved to a new city because your parents took different jobs or when you graduated from high school or from college and moved on to another phase of your life.

Many years ago, I learned a very healthy approach to relationships. Rather than getting upset if friends don't call or stay in touch, give them the benefit of the doubt by understanding that they must be busy just as I am busy. Then when we reconnect, I pick up where we left off, and in this way, I am at peace with the relationship and continue to enjoy the friendship.

We can think of our journey together like cars on a highway. We travel along the road with other cars, and then one car takes an exit and takes another road, while we journey on to our own destinations. In our lives we went to elementary school with some people and high school with others. We work with different sets of people, and our family comprises yet others. Our children are with us until they grow up, and they continue on their journeys, forming different relationships, and then they become parents with their own children.

But no matter how many journeys we take part in, our constant companions are our own body, mind, and spirit...and the rungs of the ladder also apply here.

Self-care, self-love, self-respect, self-awareness, commitment, expectation to be my best every day, being honest, and being content can allow me to have a peaceful relationship with myself.

Physical exercise, for example, helps not only the body but also the mind and spirit by reducing stress, creating a positive chemical response and releasing healthy chemicals called endorphins and balancing excess stress hormones such as cortisol.

Finally, to achieve contentment and spiritual wellness in this journey, you have to use a simple principle. If you keep your peace as your guide for every decision you make, then you continue to build a life grounded in your peace. When you go to sleep at night, all you have to do is to ask yourself one question: "Was I my best today?" If you can say yes, then go to sleep in peace. If you can't say yes, then take a moment to reflect on why not. When tomorrow comes, make it that day! To honestly be able to answer yes to this question is a key to your spiritual wellness.

As we each practice these concepts, our journey together is grounded in our peace, and we enjoy our own company as well as the company of those with whom we share this journey! As we start to find the joy in our journeys, feeling grounded in our own peace, we are able to then pay attention more fully to those around us, not just in hearing them but also in actually listening.

The true journey lies in finding peace within!

LISTENING VERSUS HEARING

This is a key factor in optimizing your relationships. The difference between listening and hearing is determined by whether you were paying attention. Listening means that you were paying attention, but hearing doesn't necessarily means the same thing. In the middle of any big city, you can hear the traffic, but at a concert, you are listening to the music. Saying, "I heard you" and showing that you're listening are two different things. Listening means that you not only heard but that you consciously, actively paid attention and that you were focused.

This gets to the heart of communication. After all, communication is one of the essential ingredients for any relationship. If both sides are talking and neither side is listening, then it leads to misunderstandings, disagreements, and ultimately, failure and dissatisfaction in the relationship. Try listening to your partners, coworkers, friends, or even people you disagree with to truly understand their perspectives or positions. Listening can lead to learning. Then when you feel like you are a good listener, listen to your "inner voice". This is the result of your conscious and subconscious working together and often reflect your core values much better than an action or decision based on emotion or sentiment.

The other important point about listening is that there are two types. There is listening with the intent to respond and listening with the intent to understand!

When I listen with the intent to respond, as soon as the other person starts speaking, I am analyzing and formulating my response. My mind is actively engaged in the response and thus is not fully engaged in the listening process. This approach causes me to be critical of the information I am receiving, and I begin to immediately filter each piece of information, ready to ping-pong an answer back.

When I listen with the intent to understand my mind is open and accepting, without judgment, supposition, or critical analysis. I allow the speaker to reveal the entirety of the "story" prior to drawing conclusions or filtering my perception with inherent bias. This is more satisfying for the narrator of the story, as he or she doesn't feel rushed or judged and can freely express without the defensive posture that people often take when they know they are going to be judged or assessed.

Listening to understand is kind and can strengthen friendships, relationships, and your own ability to see another perspective—the world through another's eyes. Listening to respond is not a bad thing, as it can be helpful when planning, organizing, building, and developing ideas. When we are able to use appropriate listening in the right setting, we create a productive and proactively positive presence. Next time someone asks you to listen, ask which type of listening he or she wishes from you. Then you don't have to guess or assume. How simple is that? *Think about it!*

Learn to listen and listen to learn.

Now: The Treasured Moment

What is it that you can have but never hold on to? It's *now*! The moment about to come just went as you thought about it, and the moment that *is* no longer is!

We all want to be there—or should I say here! Athletes call it the "zone" when they feel like they can't go wrong. At that moment they're not struggling, and everything just seems to be falling into place. They talk about "letting the game come to me rather than forcing the action!" Think about how this applies in our daily lives.

Do you have the patience to let situations in your life unfold, or do you try to force the action? Do you always feel like saying, "Come on, man! I don't have time for this! Let's go!" Are you always going hard and feeling like you hit brick walls? Are you trying to knock them down? Or do you have the patience to look for the door that opens, allowing you to move toward your goal with less stress?

Athletes who are in the "zone" are present in the moment and are not thinking about the last moment of frustration or the perceived threat around the corner. They are taking each moment and simply being present without distraction aware of the full impact and potential of the present moment—the *now* moment. This allows them to maximize the moment and their impact in it without pushing hard or struggling.

Some of us get it. Many of us don't. When standing in front of a wall and wanting to get to the other side, what are the options? One option is to break down the wall, which can be very destructive and potentially painful or harmful. Another option is to find the door and walk through to the other side, without any destruction or the consequences of that destruction. What is the difference between the two options?

The person who only sees the wall as an obstacle or problem without exploring possible solutions will feel a sense of greater frustration and may try to tear down the wall rather than find the door or straightforward solution. If you are rigid in your stance, position, or opinion and are not willing to be flexible or explore other possibilities, then you will only see the wall of obstacles and may not be flexible or patient enough to search for the doorway of solutions. What's easier—breaking down walls or walking through doors?

If you're struggling with something,
you're probably doing it wrong.

Think about it! The big decisions should not be struggles. If you're struggling with something, oftentimes it is because what you may think you want may not be what you need. Putting a square peg in a round hole, as they say, can lead to frustration. Once you find the round peg, the fit is obvious! So next time you are struggling with a decision, think about what's happening. Is your background information about the situation complete, and do you know all sides of the story? If not, then it's like having half the pieces of a jigsaw puzzle and hoping to put the whole picture together.

Take the time to inform yourself of all the known facts of a situation before jumping to conclusions or making a decision. Look at the situation from as many perspectives as you can. Then let the information brew in your mind for some time so that you can process it. With this approach you won't end up making a hasty decision that you may regret later.

To live a life with no regrets, start by making informed choices. Then as you decide what to do, remember the simple principle about choosing peace!

At every fork in the road, if you make the choice that brings you peace, then you will have a life grounded in your peace. If all of us function in this manner, then think of the wonderful possibilities.

*Peace is different for everyone, and yet the common thread
to attain it is not about getting all that you want but in
being content in having the basic things you need!*

If you're grounded in contentment, then even when you fall, you fall back to contentment. If you're grounded in discontent or dissatisfaction, then whenever you fall or something does not go your way, you fall back to that mind-set of discontent, and it can be frustrating and painful. When people don't understand this and try too hard to fill up their "bucket of wants," then they struggle more and seem to never be content. Why? Because there is always the next thing that they want!

Some people try to keep up with "the other guy" while others envy their neighbor's "green grass." This may not stress everyone but leads many people to dissatisfaction with their lives, creating unrest, anxiety, depression, hatred, remorse, or guilt. This in turn can have real biochemical and physical effects on the body.

A simple example is that when we are stressed, a chemical called cortisol goes up in the body. Cortisol is a stress hormone that has many effects, including raising blood pressure and affecting digestion, and it can even lead to long-term consequences that can affect insulin and sugar processing, body fat breakdown, immune system function, mood, the ability to fight infection and heal, bone formation and developing osteoporosis, and memory! Speaking of memory, did you already forget the first paragraph?

Yes, it happens—and oh, by the way, some of it is irreversible! People who focus on the destination and ignore the value of the journey forget that every point of the journey is a destination in and of itself.

When running a race, even though we focus on the finish line as the ultimate goal, each step along the way is a small goal that is achieved, an end unto itself. Without each step being completed, the next one cannot begin.

So take the time to be present and enjoy each step thoroughly, ensuring that when you get to the finish line, you have had a contented, satisfying, and joyful journey filled with triumphs, victories, and joyful memories to celebrate.

*In trying too hard to reach the life we want, we lose sight of
the life we are living.*

DETACHMENT

This word has deep meaning! "Attachment" means being bound to something, whereas "detachment" means not being bound to something. Detachment from the fruits of one's actions as well as detachment from negative emotions such as anger, hatred, lust, greed, depression, anxiety, and fear can lead to peace. When we are depressed or anxious, we are usually thinking about a past we can't go back and change or a possible future that isn't even a reality yet. Detachment from the past as well as the future allows us to appreciate the value of each moment. After all, tomorrow has never been guaranteed to anyone, but you have today, and you have this moment to be your best self.

Now, detachment doesn't mean you don't care about your wife, children, and parents or loved ones or that you don't get involved in their lives. It means that you detach yourself from burdening them with unreasonable or unrealistic expectations. How many of us know people who have tried to relive their childhoods through their own sons or daughters? Sometimes we are so attached to our expectations of what we individually feel *our* lives have to be or have that we don't even stop to think that others in our lives may have their own ideas. People often ask me if I *want* my son to be a doctor since I am one. I tell them that they will enjoy hearing from him what *he* wants to be! I admit I am attached to the notion that

I *do* want him to be a good person who figures out contentment, peace, love, and self-sufficiency for his life. My role is to guide him so that he may blossom and fly with his own wings and chart his path rather than try to mimic or relive mine. We can't make other people be someone they are not, and when we detach ourselves from that notion, then we can start to appreciate them for their natural qualities and beauty.

When you detach from expectations you embrace your present!

CREATING YOUR BUFFERS IN LIFE

Once when I went to a board-review course (in medicine we have to take tests called board exams every so often to certify that we are current in our knowledge), I met a retired physician who joined my colleagues and me for lunch. He must have been well past his years of active medical practice. He was quite enthusiastic to be there, and we had a great conversation with him. We asked him what he was doing at a review course. He told us that he was visiting the only family he really knew. He went on to say that as a practicing physician, between his office, nursing home care, delivering babies, and home visits, he was very busy and hardly ever home. His wife had passed away several years ago and he felt that he hardly knew his children since he had missed a great deal of their childhood due to his work schedule. His advice to us was to find the right balance of work and family time. He urged us to work enough to have enough and to make the time for family and self-care.

He pointed out the flexibility and buffering that an extra half-day or a day can give for personal and family needs. He and I also discussed the importance of budgeting that time into things like home expenses, differentiating needs and wants, and the value of creating flexibility in one's home and work routines. This has been priceless advice that has paid off time and again in my life for emotional, mental, spiritual, and physical wellness.

Put a Nickel in Every Basket

In terms of financial buffers, a simple rule to consider is to "put a nickel in every basket." I will give you an example of a teenager who wants to buy a car at age sixteen with $2000 that he has saved. He could buy the car, or he could take the $2,000 and place it in an IRA (individual retirement account). Through saving the money even just the one time, he could double that money roughly every seven years (based on past US market data and estimated 10 percent annual return). By the time he turned sixty-five, the money would have doubled seven times, equaling $256,000. Simply putting away $2,000 at age sixteen in the IRA and not touching it again would, based on the history of the financial markets over the last few decades, yield him more than a quarter of a million dollars without him doing anything else.

People often forget to put a nickel in every basket. We have to think of savings as a way of paying ourselves and creating our own bank from which we can draw money later. Simply putting as little as five or twenty-five dollars per week into a retirement account or savings account would be a start. Create separate "baskets" for the basics such as rent or mortgage, groceries, electricity, clothing, and so on. Then create separate "baskets" for nonessentials such as vacations, eating out, going to the movies, and the like. I call these nonessentials, but I should say that I believe that having fun is important. However, if you don't take care of your core needs such as food, water, and shelter, then you will have greater stress, whereas if you don't get to eat out this month, this won't be as big an issue. Get help if you need it from people who may be more financially wise! Just as importantly, take time to educate yourself so that you can be the manager of your own destiny.

This idea of placing a nickel in every basket goes well beyond finance. It can apply to relationships. Take the time to acknowledge and pay attention to all those you are in relationship with. Simple gestures are invaluable such as making eye contact, smiling, and asking people how they are and then actually listening to the response with the intent to understand.

This principle applies to the four cores of wellness themselves. Pay attention to nutrition, exercise, stress management, and your spiritual wellness. At different times in your day and in your life, different components may need a little more or a little less attention. Adjust and optimize your relationship with that component so that there is harmony and rebalancing as needed.

FINDING YOUR SPEED LIMIT

This is a reference to working and living within your comfort zone. Allow me to give you several examples.

Let's say that you and I wanted to drive to New York City from Boston. By the way, I am a proponent of the law and obeying the speed limits, but for any of you who have driven on this stretch, cars are known to travel well above the speed limit. Now, let's say that you like to drive at eighty miles per hour, and I like to drive at sixty-five miles per hour. If we were to leave at the same time and had to arrive at the same time, I may be driving out of my comfort zone to keep up with you and to meet the deadline. This could then be a source of stress and anxiety for me.

If, however, I took off from Boston an hour earlier, I could still drive within my comfort zone and arrive at my destination at the desired time and would have done so within my comfort zone without unnecessary stress or anxiety.

This reminds me of the story of the turtle and the hare. The turtle, consistently working within his comfort zone, was still able to achieve his goal.

Another simple example is that of meetings. We plan meetings but often don't plan the time to get from meeting A to meeting B. For example, let's say meeting A is at 9:00 a.m., and meeting B is at 10:00 a.m. Meeting A is supposed to last for an hour, while meeting B is across town. Well, how the heck are you supposed to get there? We don't buffer our time well, and this becomes a major source of frustration for a lot of people. Currently, we use words such as "efficiency" to symbolize how much we can pack in our schedule within a given time period. This leads to stress within the entire system.

LIVING WELL AT 80 PERCENT

This is a practical point that is as much about saving a little reserve as it is about planning for a rainy day! Can you live well at 80 percent? If you can budget so that you can live off 80 percent of what you earn then you can have a nice buffer and wise planning for the future. In America, the motto used to be that people should save at least 10 percent of their incomes for retirement. Over the last two decades, the pundits have started to tell us to save at least 20 percent of our incomes for retirement. The point is to create a buffer or a cushion so, during times of stress or unexpected shortfalls, we are not left without a reserve to draw upon.

Now if you can maintain a little reserve in terms of your emotions, relationships, and food consumption, then you will have added benefits. With food, don't overeat; be done when you feel 80 percent full. When it comes to emotions, the point is not to *not* share your feelings. Rather, think before you speak so that you don't have to feel as if you wish you could take back what you said. If your emotional response is necessary for you to have peace or you feel it will bring a positive resolution to the situation, then speak your mind. If not, then *think about it*! If what you say or do is not going to positively resolve the issue five minutes from now or five years from now, then don't stress about the situation!

> *Redefine "efficiency" to reflect how you can achieve the goal within a given time period with the least amount of stress or distress! That is efficiency for the mind, body, and spirit!*

PART 4

THE FOURTH CORE OF WELLNESS: SPIRITUAL WELLNESS

CIRCLES OF PEACE

"Spiritual wellness" can mean different things to different people. I define it here as the attainment of peace and contentment. The word "peace" also has different meanings for different people, and you have to figure out what it means for you. Once you define peace, make a plan to get to that place in your life where you have a sense of peace. Then—and this is the important but tricky part—don't let anyone take you out of this place. There will be times when you will have to figure out what is important and what is not as important to you so that you can hold onto your peace.

"Sounds very naïve," you say. You could say, "C'mon, sometimes there are more than two choices. It's not always that simple!" You'd be right, and I'm sure many people would agree. Nothing is inherently simple; we have to know how to simplify things. Break down stressful situations into basic real choices. Then we have to make a choice, and I choose peace. That doesn't mean that I would choose harm toward others, because again, as we know, that is not a choice that would lead to a peaceful end. My point is simple. When you're faced with a decision, figure out what outcome is going to bring you peace. This means you have to understand what peace means for you. Is it satisfaction, joy, happiness, being content, a combination of these, or something else? Once you figure out what peace means to you, you can keep that as your focus, and then don't lose sight of it.

We may not always be happy, but we can learn to be at
peace with any given situation.

If every decision in your life, every fork in the road, is guided by this principle of peace, then you will build a life grounded in your peace.

Peace begins within, and only then can you have peace
in the outer circles of life, such as in couplehood, with
children, parents, extended family and friends, and then
with everyone else.

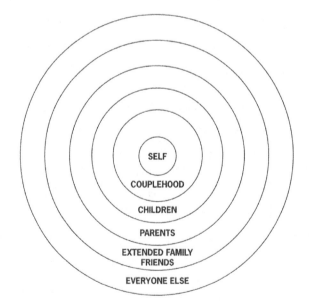

Circles of Peace

If the outer circles are affecting your inner peace, then you have to reassess your priorities. *Think about it!* Relationships are usually formed with someone else, though you also have a relationship with yourself. In each case, you are an essential part of the equation. If you are at peace, each one of your relationships has a chance to be at peace. If you are not at peace, then none of your relationships have a chance to be at peace, regardless of the others.

People talk about finding peace, attaining peace, and being at peace. We associate calm with peace. For this your breath is very important! Do the breathing exercise described in the chapter on golden light meditation to calm your mind.

You have one life with two choices. You can choose to be at peace, or you can make the other choice, but it is always your choice. Don't point the finger at anyone else!

Be at peace, for it is a choice—your choice!

Brighten Up Your Life by Getting Back to Basics

As flowers bloom, the trees blossom, and the melodious chirping of the birds signals the advent of the spring, let us nurture the joy in our hearts so that we may fertilize and sow the seeds of a life grounded in contentment and peace. This is spring cleaning of the mind, body, and spirit!

Open up the windows of your mind to let in fresh ideas and thoughts to revitalize your life, relationships, goals, and ambitions. Work off the rust, cobwebs, and baggage collected by the body during winter hibernation. Lift up your spirit by embracing all that you are and all that you can be!

So how does one find contentment and peace? I like to say that *acceptance and forgiveness lead to contentment and peace!* Brighten up your life by getting back to the basics:

1. Start by accepting yourself for who you are, imperfect and flawed, as we all are, while being unique and a one-of-a-kind original!
2. Forgive yourself if you have not always been your best to yourself. You are the only one who is with yourself 24/7/365.

3. Be nice to yourself by taking good care of your mind, body, and spirit. Follow the four cores of wellness!
4. Focus on the things you can take care of in your life, and then…guess what…start at the top of the list, and take care of one thing at a time!
5. Appreciate that you have today to create a peaceful life, and then start creating it!
6. Invite things and people into your life that will add to your joy. Be wary of things and people that take your joy away.
7. Lastly, try this simple exercise. Keep a cup on your desk at work or on the kitchen counter at home, and label it your "cup of joy." Now, every time you have a joyful moment, write it down on a piece of paper, and put it into your cup. Then, whenever you have a down moment, go to your cup of joy, pick out a slip of paper, and read it to uplift you, as that too is a real moment in your life.

Remember that if you fill your "cup of life" with joy, you have very little room for anything else! After all, if your life were a cup, would you fill it with stress, distress, anger, hatred, sorrow, greed, frustration, other negative emotions and experiences, or would you rather fill it with contentment, peace, love, and joy?

Focus on the joys, and continue to build a life full of contentment and peace by creating and collecting more joyful moments and experiences.

Connect the dots of joy in your life, and you will paint a smile!

We can all connect the other dots and paint a different picture, but why not keep on adding moments of joy in your life, and continue to connect those moments as your smile grows brighter?

CELEBRATE YOU

————⌒————

Take a few moments to look in the mirror. Do you recognize that person? Do you know that person? Do you like what you see? Are you seeing the best reflection of you?

If you answered yes to all of the above, then I'm truly happy for you! This means you are content with who you are as a person and with your life. If you were not able to answer yes, then take some time to think about why you're not. And just as importantly, ask yourself, "How can I get there?"

It all starts with understanding reality and accepting responsibility for your own life. Many people are depressed because of things that have happened in their past. They tend to blame the past for their current situations and sometimes are stuck looking in the rearview mirror! It's very hard to move forward while looking backward, wouldn't you agree?

Getting fixated on the "shoulda, coulda, woulda" prevents us from living in the now and building better futures.

Some people have a lot of anxiety worrying about an anticipated future that hasn't even occurred yet. Stuck worrying about something that may or may not happen, they lose out on the current moment. No one can predict the future, so worrying about the "what ifs" can paralyze a person into inaction. You become so concerned with the worst possible scenarios that you give up before you can even get started. You're defeated mentally and emotionally simply by the fear of something that may not even be!

As we tell athletes, "You can't win the game sitting on the sidelines!" The same principle applies in other aspects of our lives. You can't achieve much by just thinking about it; you have to make a plan and then carry it out—you have to act! If things aren't going the way you anticipated, then reevaluate and make the necessary changes so you can achieve your goals.

It all starts with being selfish enough! *Self-care, self-love, and self-respect are good types of selfishness!* Most of us are not selfish enough, and so we are unable to be our best selves!

Remember that peace begins within. Peace comes with forgiveness and acceptance. We have to forgive the past so that we may live in the present. While we can't predict the future, we can always follow the adage "Hope for the best, expect the worst, and prepare for both." Once you have done this, you will understand contentment.

Accept, adjust, and adapt!

Accept your life for what it is so that you have no delusions. Embrace it as the new starting point on your journey towards contentment and peace.

Adjust your expectations and approach situations based on who you are and what your strengths are.

Adapt to the ever-changing world we live in by paying attention to what is going on around you and to how you feel about it.

I'm not saying you shouldn't have big dreams. I'm saying you should dream big and then, in order to make it happen, know what tools you need to have in your toolbox to get the job done. Then, figure out how to get them.

Walk in your own shoes, and you will know how high you can jump, how fast you can run, how far you can go, and what effort you need to make to get to where you want to go...and then make the effort!

Look in the mirror again, and smile at the person you see...let 'em know that you love 'em...you're worth it!

The Golden Rule for Self-Care

In pursuit of happiness, one thing to remember is that if we allow happiness to be dependent on the circumstances of our lives, then it will come, and it will go! For instance, if you score the game-winning goal, you are happy, but if you get the goal scored on you, then you are not!

We can, however, learn to be at peace in life no matter what the circumstance. This begins with understanding what peace means to you and then caring enough about yourself to obtain it and maintain it.

One simple rule that will help with this is what I call the golden rule for self-care. Before getting to that, let's first relearn the golden rule.

The golden rule knows no cultural bounds. Cultures from around the world have variations of this theme. To paraphrase, it reads, "Do unto others as you would like to have others do unto you!"

Most people are aware of this rule, but how many of us consciously think about it every day? And if it is a good rule for how to treat others, then why not apply it to ourselves? That's right! This is my golden rule for self-care:

> Do unto *you* as you would like to
> have others do unto you!

This is about being *selfish*! Yes, you read that right!

Selfish is *good* when it means self-care, self-love, and self-respect. Selfishness is not good if it refers to hurting others. Most of us aren't selfish enough! A selfless man has already passed through the stage of *good* selfishness. Let's look at some great leaders of peace such as Mahatma Gandhi, Mother Teresa, and Martin Luther King. They were considered to be selfless or giving of themselves to the world. In order to become selfless, they had to find their inner peace first so that they could give of themselves to the world. Caring about yourself and aiming to become a better person is *good* selfishness.

Our eyes look out at the world around us, but we don't see ourselves! We learn that we should be considerate of the needs of others, but we also need to be considerate of our own individual needs.

If you want others to love you, then start by loving yourself! If you abuse your body or let yourself be abused in a relationship, then others will get the message that it is OK to treat you the same way. Get seven to nine hours of sleep. Do away with smoking and alcohol abuse. And *do* take time to have fun every day!

By following the golden rule for self-care, you can maintain peace and happiness in your life. By practicing self-respect, self-care, and self-love, you will also send a message to others...and they will respect you for it!

Peace and happiness do begin within.

BE LIKE WATER

When water is poured into a glass, it takes the shape of the glass, yet it still remains water. Water can take the shape of anything, and yet it still remains what it is. Water is strong enough to break down bridges and cause hurricanes and storms, and yet it is the softest substance in the world! In solid, liquid, or gas, it never loses its core propensity!

If you can be like water, then in any given situation, you can be the tsunami when you need to be or be the gentle brook. You can adapt to the situation, and yet you won't let the situation transform your core! There are times when you need to be the calm, and there are times when you need to be the storm. Sometimes you have to go with the flow, and sometimes you have to be the flow. (More on the flow as you flow into the next chapter!)

When Siddhartha Gautama, also known as the Buddha, first encountered the perils of daily life, he became frustrated and confused. You see, he was a prince, and it had been foretold to his father that Siddhartha would be a great leader or a great ruler. His father wished for his son to be a great ruler. Therefore, he isolated the prince from any negative aspects of the world outside the palace. However, one night, feeling unsettled, Siddhartha snuck out of the palace. What he saw convinced him that the life he had been living was one that lacked awareness of the realities of the world around him and not the life he wanted. He saw so much suffering all around him and began to question if there was a way to overcome suffering. He left the life that he knew in search of answers to questions regarding suffering and how to overcome it. When he felt enlightened with the knowledge of finding a path to liberation from the suffering encountered in daily living, he began teaching it to others. The title of "Buddha" means "enlightened one."

In our daily lives, we often encounter suffering, many times our own, and commonly the result of our own actions. Getting upset about a situation may be fine, but more often than not, the "getting angry" part is not going to resolve your situation. Anger is a sign of fear—something is threatening the expectation we have for a particular situation, and so we become unsettled. Anger wastes much energy and can be very powerful. The same energy, were it channeled toward pondering a solution to the problem, may become a powerful *con*structive force rather than an unpredictable *de*structive force. How many times have you seen a loved one or relative have an angry outburst only to regret it afterward because things were said or done that led to negative consequences? Think of the waters of a mighty river unleashed upon a city in its path when a dam breaks. The uncontrolled waters can wreak havoc that had not been seen when the dam was working adequately. The dam serves to guide the flow of water, just as our senses and sensibilities can serve to guide our emotions. The floodgates of a dam can be opened during times of drought to unleash the force of water, but they can also be used to harness the energy from such a powerful natural resource. If we can do that with our own energy and emotions, we are better able to guide the flow of energy and chart our course through any given situation.

Be like water and nourish your soul!

THE FLOW IS YOUR LIFE

So, what's all this talk about the flow anyway? What flow are we talking about? The flow is your life itself! So depending on the situation, you can adapt your course of action. Sometimes you have to go with the flow, and sometimes you have to lead the flow. *Think about it!*

There are times in our lives when we have to go with the flow. When things are going well in life, let the positive flow carry you along. If you're unable to see a clear path but don't see any alarming signs or red flags, go with the flow until you have a better sense of direction or until you feel you need to chart a different path. This is a time where life can be in somewhat of a cruise-control mode as you focus on strengthening your foundation and rethinking your goals.

The decision to go with the flow means you are not fighting against the current and creating turbulence in your life. This is a chance to regroup, rebuild, dream of possibilities, and choose your path to peace and contentment.

Painters talk about feeling as if the brush is guiding their hand, letting the stroke of their brush flow smoothly.

Some people find it difficult to go with the flow, and so they try to force the action and activity in their lives. Swimming against the current can be stressful and exhausting, and in the end you may find that for all your effort, you end up in the same place where you started. Remember, *if you're struggling with something, you're probably doing it wrong!* See how this applies in your life!

At other times in our lives, we have to lead the flow. When you wish to lead your children to learn good behaviors, you have to be the guiding flow leading them on the right path; lead by example. A boss has to chart the path for the flow and then can ride the wave or guide the wave as needed. When you are entering a new phase in your life or starting a new project, it's very important to be the flow and not only chart your own path but show the strength of your character and unique perspective.

To lead the flow, you have to understand the terrain. In this case, the terrain refers to the resources at your disposal, the support you have, and the hurdles in your path. Once you understand these, then it is much easier to navigate the path and lead others on it. Whenever you are choosing a direction, remember to let peace be your guide, and you will be less likely to falter.

It may be easier to go with the flow, but there are times in life when you need to lead the flow in a new direction. If your friends are smoking or using drugs, you *don't* go with the flow! If your friends are getting in the car with a drunk driver, you *don't* go with the flow. In those instances, it's best to go against the flow. When you go with the flow of who you really are, you will be naturally contented in your own flow and won't want to join in with others just because others are flowing in a different direction.

The difference between knowledge and wisdom is that the wise know when to use their knowledge. Knowledge without reflection and action leads to no change. Sometimes you have to go with the flow, and sometimes you have to lead the flow.

The flow is your life itself!

DON'T JUST DO SOMETHING: STAND THERE

My medical school years at St. George's University were spent in Grenada; Saint Vincent's; Watford, England; and the New York City and Newark, New Jersey areas in the United States. I gained some great insights during those years! One day, we were looking at x-rays of the lungs, and all of us were looking really hard and getting our noses right up to the x-ray to see if we could figure out the problem. The teaching physician took a big step back, while we all moved forward! Then he asked us what we saw.

"Mmm...uhhh...ahh...maybe some haziness over here," we said as we all pointed to different areas of the x-ray. He asked us to step back to where he was standing, and voilà—there it was. A spot that we couldn't see when we were too close was easily visible when we stepped back. It taught me that sometimes in life, we have to take a step back to be able to see things more clearly. Every so often, it is a good idea to step back and look at the trajectory of your life's path. If you are at peace and your life is maintaining the same trajectory to help you keep your peace, then continue to reinforce, nurture, strengthen, and share what you are doing. If you are not at peace or your life's trajectory is heading in a different direction, then you may want to reexamine your goals and your decisions.

The other thing I learned at the time became the title of this chapter: "Don't just do something; stand there!" The classic saying is "Don't just stand there, do something!" Some people want to react immediately when things don't seem to go their way. They hear that someone said something, and they immediately fly off the handle without getting all of the information or reflecting on the other viewpoint. When you are patient and wait for all the facts to surface and examine the situation from all sides, you have better information on which to act rather than reacting to misinformation. I would rather act based on good information than to react to misinformation. *Think about it!* Sometimes you have to let a situation sort itself out rather than trying to rush it. When you put food in a slow cooker you can't force it to get cooked faster than it will! Right?

Think about it! You're done with the book! Congratulations! You have strengthened your toolbox to help you live a life of contentment and peace. You need nothing else, for you are here in the presence of completion. Having crossed the finish line, you dwell in this place, this space that lies beyond and is inherently within you. Let love flow like a river to the sea, and let peace guide your path along the way!

May contentment and peace be our guiding light and our destination…with a little fun along the way, of course!

About the Author

Kaushal B. Nanavati, MD, is a motivational speaker and an integrative family physician in Syracuse, New York, who enjoys educating people on wellness, self-care, and achieving contentment and peace in life using humor, stories, and real, tangible examples. He has been a contributing author in local magazines and has taught end-of-life care to physicians, families, and caregivers. He was born in India and moved to Rochester, New York, at the age of seven, where he later went to high school at both Monroe and East. He then attended Rensselaer Polytechnic Institute and graduated with a degree in biology and minors in philosophy and literature. He attended St. George's University School of Medicine, and his schooling provided him experiences in Grenada; Saint Vincent's; Watford, England; and the New York City and Newark, New Jersey areas in the United States. He has worked in rural, suburban, and urban settings throughout his career, caring for all stages of life, from birth through the end of life. He has enjoyed learning karate and coaching his son in basketball, has completed a marathon, loves to play tennis and golf, and cherishes personal time with his family.

Made in the USA
Monee, IL
13 August 2021